EFT TAPPING FOR YOUR DAILY HEALTH

Use the Emotional Freedom Technique to De-Stress, Re-Energize and Overcome Emotional Problems

ZSUZSANNA T. GROUNDS

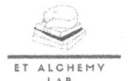

ET ALCHEMY LAB

CONTENTS

Introduction v
1. Introduction To EFT Tapping 1
2. EFT: How It Works? 7
3. EFT Basics 17
4. The Science Behind Eft 29
5. Eft Tapping Sequence 38
6. Tapping And Emotions 46
7. Gain Energy 72
8. How To You Tapping Today 77
9. Conclusions 90

INTRODUCTION

Thin Slim Consider everything like energy. Emotions and thoughts come from energy. And energy has very real physical manifestations as well.

When we experience a negative emotion, face a traumatic experience, or confront an unfavorable and unpleasant situation, excess energy is created. When this excess is not dealt with properly, over time, it can cause more serious problems. This is where the Emotional Freedom Technique (EFT) can help.

What exactly is EFT?

Developed by Gary Craig, emotional liberty is a technique of psychological acupressure that involves touching close to endpoints of the energy beams in your body. It is a powerful combination of mind and body medicine and acupressure that can help solve physical, mental, and emotional health problems. The EFT is grounded in this premise that we are more likely to be healthy and happy when free from emotional disturbances.

Numerous research studies and countless practitioners have demonstrated that EFT is very effective on several issues, including Stress, Fatigue, and Emotional issues such as low self-esteem, depression, and anxiety.

Best of all, EFT is a simple self-help technique that is easy to learn and do on your own. It's no problem to fit EFT into a busy schedule; an EFT session doesn't take long, and you can already feel better after just a few minutes.

In this book, you'll find all the information you need to learn and use this powerful self-help tool. Millions of people worldwide already use EFT for a happier, healthier, and more balanced life. I hope it will do the same for you!

Chapter One
INTRODUCTION TO EFT TAPPING

*L*et's start by looking at what tapping is and where the idea came from.

Emotional Freedom Therapy (also known as EFT) is a new psychological treatment method, an alternative therapy, widely practiced by people worldwide.

Research has shown that EFT is a very effective and efficient method that can help people in various ways.

It can help treat psychological problems like stress, anxiety and overcome addictions like smoking, drinking, gambling, etc. It can also help improve self-esteem and confidence.

EFT is based on tapping our meridian points and makes use of scripts to overcome and treat problems. You can use this powerful healing technology by taking support from a therapist or performing the techniques yourself.

EFT is a type of energy therapy and works similarly to other energy therapies, such as acupuncture and acupressure.

EFT is believed to work by rebalancing the flow of energy through the body's channels known as meridians.

Research has shown that EFT taps into a section of the brain that stores and processes data, which is used in neurophysiology.

EFT practitioners believe that negative thoughts remain as blockages in the brain, leading to a range of symptoms such as fear, anger, stress, etc.

Some of the causes behind such negative emotions include psychological or emotional disorders or events.

If you feel that you are inadequately trained, or that the trauma is too intense, or you feel that there is a lack of progress, then get in touch with a skilled competent professional who can help you to work on issues and also offer support and advice on how to improve your self-practice.

Tapping: The Origins
Emotional Freedom Therapy has its roots based on neuro-linguistic programming (also

known as NLP), behavioral kinesiology, and thought field therapy (also known as TFT).

There is an exciting story about the origin of Thought Field Therapy, which in turn paved the Emotional Freedom Therapy.

Dr. Roger Callahan was a cognitive psychologist and hypnotherapist who specialized in phobias. He was researching Chinese meridians and their effect when tapping at certain meridian points.

A patient with an acute water phobia came to see Dr. Roger Callahan. He had already tried some conventional therapies to cure her but was unsuccessful.

She complained that she often felt pain in her stomach even when she thought about water and her phobia.

Dr. Roger Callahan asked her to tap under her eyes a couple of times (this position corresponds to the stomach meridian).

By applying this seemingly simple technique, the patient was relieved of her phobia.

Later, Gary Craig, who worked with Dr. Roger Callahan in Thought Field Therapy, began applying this technique to his patients.

He improved some techniques and simplified the process, and this adapted method became Emotional Freedom Therapy.

About 5,000 years ago, the Chinese discovered a complex system involving power circuits that circulate throughout the body. These energetic circuits are called meridians. These so-called meridians are central to Eastern health practices and lay the foundation for modern acupressure, acupuncture, and other forms of healing techniques.

The energy circuits in your body cannot be seen with the naked eye. But even if you can't directly see the energy flowing, you know it's there for its effects, just like the energy in a television set. The energy flowing inside the television is not visible, but it is evident through its effects, namely the sound and image.

EFT works similarly. Perhaps you don't see it, but you can feel the energy flowing within your body. This becomes evident when you tap near the endpoints of the energy meridians in your body. Through tapping, you can feel the profound changes that occur in both your physical and emotional health. In summary, this is exactly what EFT Tapping is all about.

Western medical science focuses on the chemical nature of the human body. Until recent years, modern medical science did not recognize the subtle but powerful energy flows within and throughout the body. Over the years, however, this concept has become a popular topic of modern research.

The foundation of EFT is a combination of mind-body medicine and acupuncture. Importantly, both are backed by decades of scientific study. Even prestigious institutions, including Harvard and Stanford, among other universities, hospitals, and clinics, recognize their profound significance and effectiveness. Many scientific studies have been conducted, and some are ongoing to validate the significance of EFT Tapping concerning healing.

EFT borrows much of its healing process from the meridian system that the Chinese developed thousands of years ago. However, the difference between EFT and acupuncture is that the latter focuses primarily on treating physical ailments. On the other hand, EFT does not focus exclusively on physical ailments but also addresses and alleviates emotional problems.

In other words, EFT combines the cognitive benefits of conventional therapy with the physical benefits of acupuncture. The result is a more comprehensive treatment of both physical and emotional problems. Thus, it can be said that EFT is the emotional version of acupuncture. The biggest discrepancy between the two is EFT does not involve the use of needles.

Rather than using needles, EFT makes use of two basic processes. The first is the process of mentally "tuning in" to specific problems and individual experiences. And the other is the process of stimulating specific meridian points throughout the body. This is done by touching these points with the fingertips. EFT is properly administered and applied, it can help balance energy flow and eliminate disturbances in the meridian system.

Chapter Two
EFT: HOW IT WORKS?

The emotional freedom technique uses acupressure and psychology to help improve a person's emotional health.

Although emotional health tends to be overlooked, it plays a crucial role in a person's physical health and healing ability.

Never mind how dedicated we are to maintain a proper lifestyle and diet, if they have emotional barriers standing in their way, they will not achieve the body they want.

Most of the time, you can apply EFT directly to your physical symptoms to find relief without working through emotional contributors. However, you need to understand and work through the emotional issues for a powerful and lasting result.

The premise of EFT also includes that the more emotional issues you can resolve, the more emotional peace and freedom you will have.

With EFT, you can get rid of limiting beliefs, increase personal performance, improve relationships, and improve physical health. To be honest, everyone on Earth has a couple of emotional issues that they are holding onto.

EFT is extremely easy to learn and can help you in areas such as:

- achieving positive goals
- eliminating or reducing pain
- reducing
- food cravings, and
- removing negative emotions.

And that's just the beginning of what it can do for you.

EFT is based on the energy meridians that have been used in traditional acupuncture to heal emotional and physical problems for more than five thousand years, but without using needles.

Instead, it uses the simple touch of your fingertips to move kinetic energy into a specific meridian as you think about your problem and speak an affirmation.

The use of affirmations and meridian touch help clear emotional blockage from the bioenergetic system. This then helps to restore the balance of body and mind necessary for optimal health.

Many are wary of this practice at first, mainly thoughts of electromagnetic energy flowing through the body.

Then others are taken aback by thoughts of how EFT tapping works.

You need to understand that with this technique, you are touching with your fingers. Several acupuncture meridians live on your fingertips, so when you tap, you are using the energy in your fingertips and the energy of the area you are tapping.

Traditionally tapping is done by the index and middle fingers and with only one hand. You can use any hand you want.

Many of the tapping points are on both sides of the body, so that means you can use any side you want, and you can switch sides during a tapping session.

You can also modify your practice by using all fingers and hands to create a gentle, natural curved line. The more fingers you use, the more acupuncture points you'll have access to.

You'll also cover more area so you can hit the points more easily than with a pair of fingers. It's also important to take off any bracelets or watches you might be wearing.

Affirmation statements

Another important part is finding the affirmation statement you will use.

Traditionally, the statement is something like, *"Even though I have this (fill in the blank), I accept myself deeply and completely."*

You should fill in the blank with a brief description of the negative emotion, food craving, addiction, or other issues you are experiencing.

You can also use the following variations. All of the following are great to use because they use the same basic format. This means that they recognize what the problem is and create acceptance despite the existence of the problem. These are the things that are important in creating an effective statement.

The traditional one is easier to remember, but feel free to use one of the following.

"I accept myself even though I (fill in the blank)," or *"Even though I (fill in the blank), I accept myself deeply and profoundly."*

You can also use *"I accept and love myself even though I (fill in the blank)."*

Some interesting facts about affirmations are:

- you don't have to believe that you affirm; all you have to do is say it.
- It's more effective if you can say it with emphasis and feeling, but just saying it will still do the job.
- It's best to speak it out loud, but if you're in public where you have to mumble or do it quietly, it will be just as effective.

You can tune into your problem by simply thinking about what it is.

If you don't tune into your problem, which creates energy disruptions, then EFT will not be effective.

Advice and caution

You should always only do what feels right for you. Never enter physical or emotional waters that could be threatening.

It is your job to make sure you stay safe in this environment. You can easily seek professional assistance if needed.

Here are some tips before you dive into EFT:

1. It is extremely important that you are super-specific with your language when using EFT
2. You need to be completely tuned into your problem. If you are dealing with something very painful, you will try to disconnect from your feelings.
3. Because you are working with energy, it is important to pay attention to a cognitive shift. You'll know when one has happened because it reframes the problem.
4. When you see the problem from a different perspective, you will likely be surprised or new insight. This is great when this happens and can open up new and valuable insights.
5. Make sure you stay well hydrated. Water helps conduct electricity, and you are accessing electricity when you practice EFT.

Range of EFT applications
The only thing that can limit what EFT can do for you is your imagination.

Experienced practitioners and creators of EFT

around the world, including psychotherapists and psychologists, have used EFT on various issues.

This means that they have used it not only with emotional issues, where it works best but also for physical issues, with amazing success, whenever there is an emotional component or a related traumatic experience.

But that's not the only thing; EFT is also a great tool for personal development. It can help eliminate self-imposed restrictions that prevent people from experiencing abundance, great relationships, wealth, and happiness in their lives.

In EFT's short history, it has already been able to help over a thousand people with many common emotional issues, including issues such as:

- confusion, grief, guilt, and just about every other emotion you can imagine
- insecurity
- the child's inner problems and negative memories
- all kinds of phobias and fears
- depression
- frustration and anger
- anxiety and stress

What is surprising is that the advantages are not end

there. EFT tapping isn't just limited to getting rid of painful emotions.

It can also help improve your health:

- increase feelings of well-being
- help with insomnia
- relieve feelings of pain
- reduce physical cravings, for example, for chocolate and cigarettes

It can improve your effectiveness in the things you do, including:

- giving you the confidence to speak in front of a crowd and with people you are unable to communicate with at the moment
- improving personal and business relationships
- Improving your performance in sports, work, and any other area of your life

Improve the quality of your life, too:

- fostering spiritual and personal growth
- giving you the courage to try things you wanted to but were afraid to do

- Removing blocks that have kept you from having a life full of love and joy

There are many examples of people who could easily recover from emotions that had been bothering them for years, and sometimes decades, with the use of EFT.

It was something that people could turn to for help when nothing else was able to help them.

It has also successfully helped to read various physical systems such as insomnia, back pain, and headaches.

The power of EFT is at its best when the physical symptoms are also related to anxiety and stress.

EFT developers had reported an 80-100% success rate when dealing with emotional issues. When it comes to physical ailments, the success rate is slightly lower.

Most of the time, the effects of EFT are permanent, and if they are not, you can easily repeat the process if needed.

It works quickly and is gentle. People can often release emotions like stress, anger, anxiety, and fear in one session, a few days, or a couple of weeks compared to months or years of traditional therapy.

One of the best things about EFT is the fact that it is so versatile. When you master the skills it takes, which aren't difficult, it's almost like developing your superpowers.

You can use these tools in virtually any situation. For example, if you have a big presentation to give at work, or you're going in for a job interview, you can use EFT right beforehand to help calm your nervousness. It doesn't require anything special, but it works wonders and can be used anywhere.

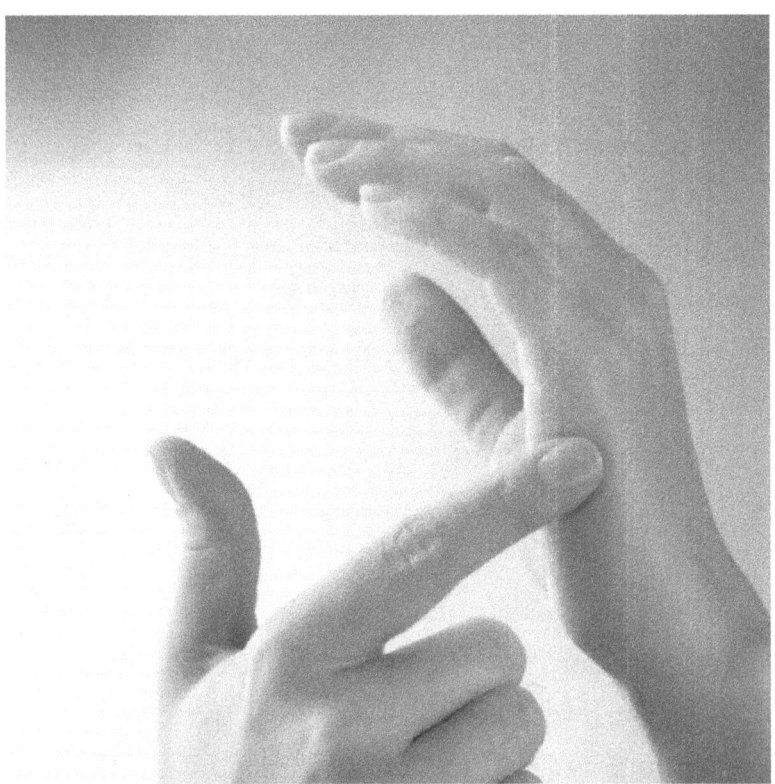

Chapter Three
EFT BASICS

Emotional Freedom Technique founder Gary Craig has developed a basic recipe for applying EFT Tapping. This recipe includes five basic steps:

- Step 1: Identify the problem
- Step 2: Assessing the problem
- Step 3: The set-up
- Step 4: The tapping sequence
- Step 5: Tuning for Re-evaluation

STEP 1: IDENTIFY THE PROBLEM

The first step is to identify the problem, issue, or emotion you want to work on. What is bothering you? Use it as a destination to be addressed during the touch session. You need to give it a name. For example, if you struggle with a bad temper, state it this way, "I find it difficult to control my temper."

By naming the problem, you focus and turn your attention to it, along with the energetic disruptions this problem creates. For the EFT session to be effective, you need to address one problem at a time.

Now, if you find it difficult to tune into the problem, or if it is too painful to think about, it may be a better idea to seek professional help rather than running EFT as a self-help tool. If you're dealing with a particularly difficult problem like depression, it's important to examine the problem one layer at a time.

Work on the surrounding issues before diving deep into the problem. Don't start with emotional problems that are too threatening to handle on your own. It can hurt more than it helps.

STEP 2: ASSESS THE PROBLEM

After identifying the problem you want to work on, it's important to rate the problem. Rate it on a scale of 0 to 10, with 0 being no problem whatsoever and ten being the worst. This rating serves as a comparison of how you feel about the problem before and after the touch rounds. It serves as a measure of how helpful EFT is for your case.

When dealing with emotional issues, founder Gary

Craig recommends reliving memories and replaying them in your mind to help you assess the discomfort or displeasure you feel about the issue.

When assessing the issue at hand, it is helpful to ask questions. How intense is the displeasure you feel because of the problem on a scale of 0 to 10? How angry does it make you think about the problem? How much do you want to work on or resolve this issue? How anxious does it make you feel? These types of questions will further help you place the problem on the intensity scale.

STEP 3: CONFIGURATION

To perform configuration, you must first draft a statement that focuses on the problem you want to solve. Through the configuration statement, you need to acknowledge the problem. At the same time, the statement must be followed by a self-affirming statement. With this structure, you engage exposure therapy and cognitive therapy simultaneously by tuning in to the problem and voicing positive affirmations about the specific problem you are addressing.

The basic structure of setup instruction is similar to the same:

- "Even though _____ (I state the

identified problem), I accept myself deeply and completely."
- The following are examples of setup instructions:
- *"Even though I find it difficult to control my temperament, I accept myself deeply and completely."*
- *"Even though I find it difficult to fall asleep, I accept myself deeply and completely."*
- *"Even though I am stressed about work, I accept myself deeply and completely."*
- *"Even though I find it difficult to connect with my family, I accept myself deeply and completely."*
- *"Even though I am often irritated with my spouse, I accept myself deeply and completely."*

As you tune in and focus on the problem, you may find it difficult to believe in the affirmation. However, these affirmations are important, as they help develop self-acceptance. They are instrumental in the process of learning to accept yourself for all that you are. Although saying the statements repeatedly is enough, preferably say them with conviction if you can.

The setup statement is meant to allow the emotion

to be free from resistance and self-rejection simply. The self-acceptance statement with tuning in and assessing the intensity of the problem brings it into the present moment. It makes the problem and the emotion real.

With this structure of the EFT process, the emotion can be safely expressed and felt. This is because a clear distinction is made between the unacceptability of the problem and complete and unconditional acceptance of oneself.

In the setup phase, only one touchpoint is used. This is the karate cutting point, the part of the hand that is used to make karate chops. It is the fleshy part on the outer side of the palm, between the wrist and the child's finger.

Say the setup statement aloud while gently touching (with two or more fingers) on the karate chop spot on your hand. If you cannot say the statement aloud because you are in the company of others, simply say the words silently to yourself.

Repeat the setup instruction at least three times as you continue to touch the karate cut point. You may stop after three repetitions, but you are free to continue until you feel completely comfortable. Do you feel relaxed and ready to continue? Then let's move on to step 4!

STEP 4: TAP SEQUENCE

After finishing the setup phase, we will begin with

the tapping sequence. We will touch the following eight key meridian points:

1. Beginning of the eyebrow - Between the top of the nose and the beginning of the eyebrow.
2. Side of the eye - The bony part on the outside of the eye, near the temple.
3. Under the eye - The bone under the eye, on the top of the cheek.
4. Under the nose - Between the nose and the upper lip.
5. Chin - The indentation located between the lower lip and the chin.
6. Below the collarbone - Just below the collarbone, about two inches from the midpoint of the body.
7. Under the arm - Found on the side of the body, this meridian point is about four inches below the armpit. It's on a par with the nipple for men. And for women, it is in the middle of the bra strap.
8. Top of the Head - The highest point on the top of the head.

For a better reference, refer to the map below:

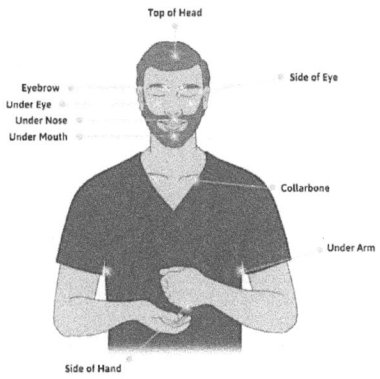

As you can see in the maps, some touchpoints are mirrored on both sides of the body. It doesn't matter if you touch the EFT or right side of the body, as long as you keep it consistent.

To get the tapping technique right, apply firm but gentle pressure. Do it as if you were tapping your fingertips on a desk. Remember to use your fingertips and not your fingernails. When touching the three largest areas, i.e., the collarbone, top of the head, and under the arm, you can use two or more fingers, depending on your preference. However, when touching the other meridian points, it is important to use only two fingers, preferably the middle and index fingers. This is because these tapping points are smaller and more sensitive areas.

Touch each meridian point in the sequence indicated, beginning with the inside of the eyebrow and ending on the top of the head. You work to stimulate your body's energy system by touching these points, thus encouraging harmony and balance.

But tapping alone is not enough; it is also important to utter a reminder phrase. This phrase indicates the problem at hand. It is the first and negative part of your configuration statement. For example, if your set-up statement is *"Even though I find it difficult to control my temperament, I accept myself deeply and completely,"* then your reminder phrase is "I find it difficult to control my temperament." You can also simply say, "I feel _____ (states the emotion, problem or issue)."

The purpose of this phrase is to keep your focus on the problem at hand. Conventional therapies avoid negative statements. On the other hand, EFT treats the focus on the negative as an essential part of releasing the problem, issue, or negative emotion.

The tapping sequence, however, should not end with negative phrases alone. The second and subsequent rounds of tapping should highlight positive affirmations, suggesting that it is possible to overcome the problem.

For the second and subsequent rounds of tapping, say a positive phrase as you touch each meridian point. Below are some examples you can refer to.

"I believe in my ability to change and solve this problem."

"I am glad to know that I can feel calm about this emotion."

"I feel joy about these positive changes."

"I am choosing to feel relaxed despite this problem."

" I'm pleased because I want to accomplishing so much."

"It feels good to be free of this negative emotion."

"I'm enjoying the peace and calm that I have right now."

"I like knowing that I have found a solution to my problem."

"I love, respect, and appreciate the person I am."

"I am more relaxed and joyful now."

" I choose to release negative emotions."

Always speak up when you are touching, as this will keep your mind focused on the problem. In public places or the company, just say the words quietly to yourself.

It's up to you how many rounds of tapping you do in your EFT session. Keep tapping until you feel more relaxed.

STEP 5: TUNE IN AND RE-VOTE

For the final part of the EFT exercise, you will be asked to review the problem. Tune in to how you feel after the touch session. Rate it from 0 to 10.

Do you still feel the same intensity? Does the

problem still make you feel as angry? Do you still feel the same level of anxiety thinking about it? Rate how you feel now and go back to your rating in Step 1. Is there any difference?

If you feel like you haven't reached the result you are looking for, keep tapping. Just go back to the configuration step in Step 3 and start tapping again from there. Update your configuration statement according to how you feel now, for example, by saying something like, "I'm releasing this remaining stress."

You can continue tapping until:

- The intensity of the problem reaches 0, or
- The intensity of the problem stops decreasing.

In some cases, repeated and continuous tapping may be necessary, especially when dealing with deeply rooted emotional problems. If there is no significant change, improve your methods. Try different things. Improve your sentences. Relax and focus more. But if you feel that the problem is not improving further or being resolved satisfactorily, you can stop touching the problem and move on to other things you want to work on.

To summarize, here are the five basic steps to EFT tapping:

- Step 1: Identify the problem - tune in and identify the issue, problem, or emotion.
- Step 2: Rate the problem - What is the intensity level of your problem? Rate it on a scale of 0 to 10, with 0 being no problem whatsoever and ten being the worst.
- Step 3: Configuration - Based on the problem you want to solve, draft a configuration statement with the following structure: "Although _____ (state the identified problem), I deeply and completely accept myself." Continue to touch the karate cut point on the outside of your palm as you say your set-up statement out loud at least three times.
- Step 4: Touch Sequence - Touch the eight meridian points in the recommended sequence as you say the reminder statement aloud. For the first round of touching, use your problem as the reminder phrase. For example, "I feel very stressed." For the second and subsequent rounds of tapping, say statements

in the form of positive affirmations, suggesting that you can overcome the problem. For example, "I choose to feel calm and relaxed."
- Step 5: Tune in and reassess: tune in and reassess the problem on a scale of 0 to 10. If necessary, return to Step 3 and continue tapping. Update your configuration instruction based on how you feel now. Continue tapping until the intensity of the problem reaches 0 or stops decreasing.

Chapter Four

THE SCIENCE BEHIND EFT

*E*FT tapping is based on the centuries-old meridian system of healing introduced by the Chinese.

Acupuncture and acupressure, which are forms of meridian system healing, are now accepted healing techniques validated by acclaimed scientific institutions such as Harvard, Stanford, and other major universities and prestigious hospitals worldwide.

In a sense, since acupuncture and acupressure have already gained acceptance as a healing technique, we can say if EFT tapping should. After all, EFT tapping is a form of acupressure and acupuncture based on the healing meridian system.

If you want more evidence on the authenticity and effectiveness of EFT tapping, you just need do some

Internet search, and you will find a wide range of scientific studies conducted on EFT tapping.

In a 2012 study on the effects of EFT on stress, subjects were randomly assigned to an emotional freedom technique (EFT) group, a psychotherapy group receiving supportive interviews (SI), or a no-treatment (NT) group.

The EFT group showed statistically significant improvements in anxiety and depression than the group that received no treatment and showed lower levels of the stress hormone cortisol.

In another study investigate whether Thought Field Therapy (also known as EFTT) could impact a variety of anxiety disorders. Forty-five patients were randomly assigned to EFTT or a waitlist control group.

Patients assigned to the EFTT treatment group showed a significant decrease in all symptoms.

More interesting, however, was that the significant improvement seen after treatment was still evident the following year, demonstrating that EFTT can have a lasting anxiety-reducing effect.

A 2013 study set out to assess the short-term effects of EFT on sufferers of tension-type headaches. Patients were randomly assigned to one of two groups. Those in the EFT group reported a significant reduction in the frequency and intensity of headache episodes.

It's early days for the science behind EFT, but of course, it was only a few decades ago that acupuncture and acupressure were also considered strange alternative therapies.

If you want to determine how useful EFT tapping is, the best way is to give it a test and start practicing it.

You yoursel best measure of how effective an EFT tapping healing technique is for your emotional issues.

The first statement of discovery, emotional healing

The philosophy behind EFT tapping can be summed up in one statement:

The cause of all negative emotions is the disruption of the body's energy system.

EFT tapping practitioners disagree with the conventional psychotherapy practice to relieve traumatic memory repeatedly so that the person heals from their negative emotional effects.

EFT tapping believes it is necessary to recognize the memory to heal. However, it is more important to identify how and wherein the memory or experience has disrupted the body y system.

Healing should be focused more on identifying the pressure point in the Meridian system that has been interrupted and applying EFT tapping techniques on a said pressure point to get the energy flowing as it normally does.

The second breakthrough statement: physical relief

EFT can aid physical healing by resolving underlying energetic or emotional contributors.

EFT practitioners understand that not all physical ailments require tapping into emotional triggers for EFT tapping techniques to heal them.

This is because some physical ailments are simply caused by a disruption in the balance of energy flow in the system. They are not caused by emotional stress or trauma.

When this happens, healing the physical ailment will only require touching the particular pressure point without focusing the mind on an emotional catalyst.

Some physical ailments are so basic that all it requires is tapping the point in the body where the energy circuit is located.

When using EFT tapping to heal the body, mind, and spirit, it is necessary to distinguish between illness caused by emotional stress or a simple physical disruption of energy flow in the body's meridian system.

The reason for this is that EFT tapping healing techniques differ depending on the disorder. Is it caused by emotional trauma or a physical disruption of energy flow?

To be effective, make sure you can identify between

the two so you can identify the most effective EFT tapping technique for healing.

EFT tapping points: the energy meridian

To practice EFT tapping and enjoy its health benefits, you must first understand the EFT tapping points or the energy meridian located throughout the body.

Below you will find a list of EFT tapping points; they are the locations of the ends of the energy meridian and are located just under the skin.

These EFT tapping points are very sensitive to touch. These same tapping points are used by acupressure and acupuncture to bring healing and physical ease to the body.

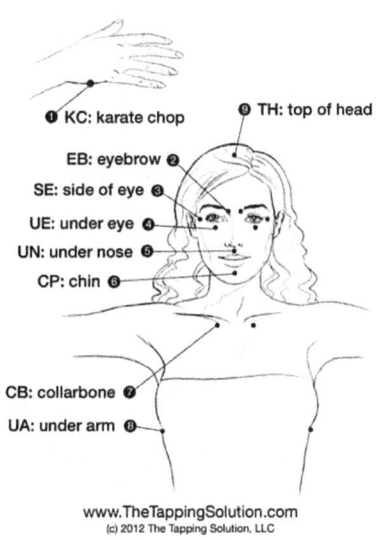

Here are the locations of the EFT intercept points:

1. The top of the head or also known as the steering vessel
2. The beginning of the eyebrow or the bladder meridian
3. The sore spot or the neuromyopathic point
4. The side of the eye or the gallbladder meridian
5. Under the eye or the stomach meridian
6. Under the nose or the ruler's vessel
7. The chin or the central vessel
8. The beginning of the clavicle or renal meridian
9. Below the nipple or liver meridian
10. The Karate Chop or the small intestine meridian
11. The baby finger or the heart meridian
12. The middle finger or the heart protector
13. The index finger or the large intestine meridian
14. The thumb or the pulmonary meridian
15. Under the arm or the spleen meridian

Each of these tapping points is connected to a specific, key organ of the body. This means that the body's organs are the points in the energy circuit where energy flows to keep the body healthy.

You might want to learn something and memorize which organ of the body each EFT touchpoint is connected to. This way, you will be able to focus on the EFT point to heal the particular part of the ailing body.

For example, if you have a migraine, it might be helpful to touch the EFT points located in the head area for immediate relief.

If you're looking for complete, long-term healing, it's best to cover all 15 EFT touchpoints in one session. In the same way that a full body massage, or a full-body acupressure session, brings full relief to the entire body, mind, and soul, a full-bodied EFT tapping session can have the same complete release of tension and stress throughout the body.

Some people find the EFT tapping point below the nipple a bit of an awkward spot to cover. It is okay to skip this part during the EFT touch session. But it can come in handy when you have health issues to deal with that affect the liver meridian. When you do this, it is necessary to touch the EFT touchpoint below the nipple.

A special EFT touchpoint not included in the list is called Gamut. It is located in the back of both hands and is behind and between the knuckles right at the base of the ring finger. It is an important EFT tapping point connected to the heart, lungs, and liver.

Come on, stand by the mirror and locate all 16 EFT touchpoints.

You must first familiarize yourself with where each touchpoint is located. This is a good and necessary start to practicing EFT tapping techniques.

How do I start tapping?

Let's take a look at how you begin to touch.

When you touch the karate hood point, which is the side of your hand (on the side opposite your thumb), use all four fingers of your other hand.

When you touch your face, use your index and middle fingers together to touch the skin gently.

When touching the collarbone, you can use the palm of your hand.

Remember, you are about to touch bony areas. To give you an idea, here's a typical routine you might follow for a touch round:

Eyebrow - touch from the inner edge of the eyebrow, above the bridge of your nose, then move to the side of the eye (between the outer edge of the eye and the hairline) - touch here, moving until you are touching under the eye (below the pupil of the eye, just around the corner cheekbone) - tapping gently with two fingers under the nose (from the back of the nose to the upper lip) - tapping gently on the chin (on the crease between the lip and the chin) using two fingers.

Then move to the collarbone, using the palm to touch under the arm (about one hand width below the armpit), touch using four fingers or the palm.

Finish by touching the top of the head, using only two fingers.

This is what you will do, for each round of touch, as you say the words, which we will see later.

Typically, you will go through several rounds of touch while:

- Express the problem
- Understand the problem
- Explore the possibilities and what you might change or do
- Relax - start using positive, calming words
- Slow down - express how you can slow down
- Choose calm and peace - affirm the positive

Chapter Five

EFT TAPPING SEQUENCE

The EFT Heart and Soul Tapping sequence

Another tapping sequence is called the Heart and Soul *EFT tapping sequence*

The Heart and Soul tapping sequence is a great alternative and just as easy to use as the classic EFT tapping sequence. My recommendation would be to try both to see which one you find more comfortable and effective.

What makes this tapping sequence different?

It's not just about tapping or touching points. The conscious mind plays a special role in this energy work. The mind has a huge impact on whether an EFT session works or not. If you unconditionally embrace the concept that EFT is about working with energy, you can get a better result from EFT. Otherwise, practical blocks may occur.

The Heart and Soul protocol was developed to address these possible practical blockages that can disrupt a smooth flow of energy. When such disturbances are eliminated, every round of tapping can produce the best results. It will lead to a maximum increase in energy flow. This tapping protocol or sequence is designed with energy at its core.

There are seven main differences between the Heart and Soul protocol and the classic EFT protocol:

1. *Heart Healing Posture*

Begin the Heart and Soul touching sequence by placing both hands in the center of your chest. This posture helps you connect with the center of your body's energy system. In this way, you can speak your set-up statement in a more conscious and focused way. It is especially helpful if you are performing EFT with a healing intention.

The heart-healing posture is also performed at the end of the tapping sequence to bring more attention to the treatment and end it with the practitioner feeling centered and grounded. It also encourages cognitive insights, which can be very valuable.

1. Top of Head

The crown point consists of various energy inputs and outputs. It serves as a central power channel for the body's energy system. This point is particularly effective in treating different types of addictions, and as a true energy point, it can help with many other things as well.

The classic protocol also touches the crown point, but the difference is that instead of ending with the crown point, the heart and soul touch sequence puts it at the beginning. From the top of the head, everything moves down the body to other treatment points, following gravity. Because of this, some practitioners believe this sequence is more natural.

1. Third Eye Point

The third eye point (the center of the forehead) is left out on the classical protocol. However, it is essential in the Heart and Soul protocol because the third eye point represents global consciousness. It is a representation of spirituality.

To touch the third eye is to invoke higher powers for assistance in the process of healing and change and ask our higher selves to be involved and more responsive during the session. Adding this point to the sequence provides a more rounded form of self-healing in EFT.

1. Axillary point eliminated

The Heart and Soul touch sequence drops the underarm point simply because some people may find it out of place or have difficulty locating the exact point to touch.

1. Finger points

The Heart and Soul protocol also includes touch-points on all five fingers. These points can allow blocked energy to flow out of the body.

1. Emphasis on Breathing

Breathing is an essential part of the Heart and Soul tapping sequence. It is meant to help release stress and relax the practitioner. The right breathing technique can go a long way in improving energy flow.

The Heart and Soul Touching sequence incorporates deep breathing into the exercise at the beginning and during the sequence. Taking a nice deep breath as you move from one point to the next can aid in creating rhythm, which is stabilizing and helps energy flow.

7. Set-up Statement

For the set-up statement, the phrase "I deeply and

completely accept myself" is optional. Especially for beginners, this last part of the set-up statement can be difficult if they don't believe in it, which may reduce the effectiveness of the EFT session.

In the Heart and Soul protocol, you simply state the problem in your own words as briefly as possible. So, if you are dealing with a lot of stress, your set-up statement would simply be something like, "I have a lot of stress." Paying attention only to the actual problem at hand ensures that the EFT session stays focused and doesn't get caught up in other problems.

How the EFT heart and soul tapping sequence is done

1. The Heart Center - To begin the tapping round, assume the heart healing posture. Place both hands flat on your chest. Take a deep breath and slowly exhale. Do this three times.
2. Top of Head - Speak your set-up statement and begin tapping the crown point. Inhale and exhale deeply before moving from one

treatment point to the next. Repeat the set-up statement at each touchpoint.

3. Third eye point - This point is located in the center of the forehead.
4. Beginning of the eyebrow - Between the top of the nose and the beginning of the eyebrow.
5. Wedge of the eye - On the bone with the corner of the eye.
6. Beneath the eye - On the bone below the eye, in line with the pupil, if looking straight ahead.
7. Under the nose - Between the nose and the upper lip.
8. Under the mouth - The indentation that is between the lower lip and the chin.
9. Under the collarbone - This point is located at the angle formed by the sternum and collarbone.
10. Thumb - All finger points are located on the finger side, in line with the nail bed.
11. Index finger
12. Middle finger
13. Ring finger
14. Little finger
15. Karaté Chop Point – Sideways the hand.

16. The Heart Center - To end the tapping sequence, return to the heart healing position. Pause for a moment to reflect. Breathe in and out three times, deeply and slowly.

Notice that you keep repeating the setup instruction at each touchpoint. So, in this exercise, the reminder statement is the same as your setup statement. This ensures that it is clear what problem you are working on at all times. So, if your problem is "I have a lot of stress," that will be your setup statement and reminder phrase throughout the session.

The map below illustrates all the touchpoints of the Heart and Soul protocol.

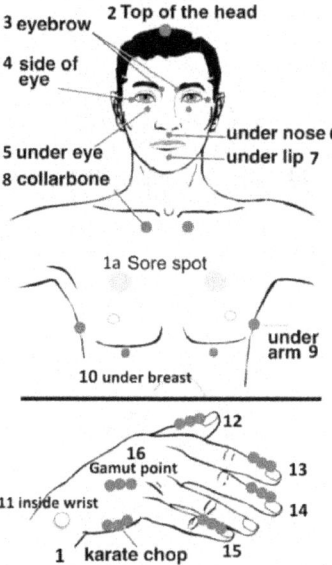

EFT - Emotional Freedom Technique
Tapping Points

You have now learned how to do EFT Tapping, using either the classic EFT protocol or the Heart and Soul protocol. You can choose which one you find more comfortable and effective, but you can also use them interchangeably if you wish.

Chapter Six
TAPPING AND EMOTIONS

The EFT is a strong tool that can help understand more about yourself, your strengths, your weakness. It can help you cope with emotions and improve relationships.

Before we begin, let me remind you that this book is not intended to substitute for doctors' medical advice.

The reader or listener should consult a physician regularly in matters related to his or her health, especially as it relates to symptoms that may require medical diagnosis or treatment.

Relationship issues

A fundamental requirement of every human being is to be loved.

When someone feels neglected and unloved, it naturally creates relationship problems, depression, and low self-esteem.

Of course, we tend to be attracted others who have similar personality traits.

For example, if you value honesty, you are more likely to attract and be attracted to an honest person. If you love yourself, then you are more likely to meet and attract others to you.

However, if you hate yourself, you create barriers that prevent others from approaching you and entering your life. Negative feelings like jealousy can seriously damage personal relationships and need to be addressed.

Suppose you feel jealous or harbor negative thoughts about yourself or your partner. In that case, likely, these thoughts or feelings are also hurting your relationship.

The first step in dealing with those problems is to do so take ownership of them.

If you are having trouble getting close to someone, want to leave a relationship, cope with jealousy, anger, or another negative emotion, you can follow the steps below.

Tap the script for relationship problems

Below are examples of setup scripts that you can use

for the touch procedure. Feel free to modify them to fit and reflect your needs.

Even though I am afraid of getting close, I accept my flaws and myself and would be able to overcome these issues.

Even though I have been in abusive relationships, I accept that I can be a better partner and master courage.

Even though I dispose of it, I love and accept myself completely.

Next, touch your energy meridian points, starting with the karate chop point and then moving downward from your head as you network your sentence.

Repeat the process and check how good you feel. Do you feel less jealous? Are you more comfortable in the relationship? If necessary, you can repeat the process.

How to deal with personal differences in a relationship

When you're in a relationship, there's often a big personal issue that arises that you'll need to heal, both for you and your partner.

Spending quality time together and talking openly about personal differences can help you overcome some of the obstacles in the relationship.

Tap to address personal differences in a relationship

You both need to sit down together and list the good qualities you like in your partner.

Then, jot down the qualities you don't like in your partner. I am aware that this will be difficult, but it is better, to be honest.

Then, write down what all the experiences in your relationship made you feel happiest (like surprise gifts).

Now, speak to your partner about what you write down, emphasizing your good qualities and being honest about the bad.

Formulate setting phrases such as "Even though I'm lonely when she's at work, I know she loves me" or "Even though we fight, I know she loves me."

I think that's good practice to start with a more insignificant issue.

You can end the process by touching together. You can also use touch scripts such as "We love each other and will work on our flaws together."

Stress

Stress is considered the slow and silent killer. Its effects on the body not only reduce your mood but can compromise your immune system.

Science has shown that stress can reduce life expectancy and is becoming a bigger problem, affecting more and more people every day.

Today, one of the leading causes of stress is work, leading to anxiety and depression, and stress.

By effectively using EFT in your daily life, you can combat stress.

Here are some benefits of using EFT and touch to cope with stress:

you can feel more motivated and more easily able to achieve your goals

Perhaps you're in a better position to deal with your anger issues.

you may become more able to adapt to different situations

you may be able to work better with your colleagues and clients

Now, let's check out a practice way to put this into action.

Taping Routine for Stress

Say these phrases as you touch the karate chop point of your hand:

Even if I feel overwhelmed by the number of things I have to do, I will find peace and clarity.

Although problems will arise if I don't finish soon, this unnecessary stress makes me feel overwhelmed and want to find peace.

Even though I have many things to do, I can be more mindful from now on about what I commit to and what I delegate.

Touch the points on your body as you say the

sentences on the right out loud.

Case 1: Express Overpowering

Top of the Head

I have so much to do!

Eyebrow

I feel so overwhelmed!

Side of Eye

How am I supposed to do everything?

Under the eye

I can't believe how much I have to do

Under the nose

I feel like I had to climb a huge mountain

Chin

It looks like I'll never be able to climb to the top

Collarbone

There's so much to do that I don't even know where to start

Under the arm

I'll be able to start once I have some clarity

EFT Round 2: Understanding overwhelm

Top of Head

I can think much more clearly when I'm not feeling pressured

Eyebrow

My head feels like it's spinning from the number of tasks I have to do

Side of Eye

This is not life or death. Where does the urgency come from?

Under the eye

Not all of these tasks are urgent

Under the nose

Some of them need to be done now

Chin

Some of them can be done later

Collarbone

Only some of them are urgent

Underarm

Worrying about everything at the same time is nonsense

EFT Round 3: Exploring the Possibilities

Top of Head

Just creating more pressure on myself

Eyebrow

Would it be good if everything came together?

Side of the eye

Like pieces of a puzzle?

Under the eye

Without me having to stress

Under the nose

Maybe I can prioritize the tasks

Chin

So the most important ones get done

Collarbone

I can handle those

Under the arm

And feel good about accomplishing something important

EFT Round 4: Relaxing

Top of head

If I focus only on the important things

Eyebrow

So I can reduce the feeling of overwhelm

Side of the eye

Because this feeling is affecting me negatively

Under the eye

And reduce my ability to work

Under the nose

Which is only taking me away from my goal

Chin

I'm smart enough to prioritize things

Collarbone

I'm going to slow down and focus

Under Arm

And create an effective to-do list

EFT Round 5: Slowing Down

Top of head
I just need to slow things down
Eyebrow
No running through everything
Side of the eye
Things will happen when I am calm and have clarity
Under the eye
There is great power in being clear about
Under the nose
Knowing what needs to be done
Chin
I will now slow down and concentrate
Collarbone
This stress is not helping me
Underarm
I have more control when I'm calm and relaxed

EFT Round 6: Choosing Peace and Calmness
Top of Head
I choose to release this stressful energy
Eyebrow
And focus on doing the things I can do now
Side of the eye
I am letting go of this overwhelming feeling
Under the eye
I choose to have a clear mind

Under the nose

I feel more relaxed and focused

Chin

With every breath, I take in and out

Collarbone

I choose to feel good knowing that I am smart and responsible

Under Arm

I choose to feel calm, confident, and powerful

As before, feel free to adjust the wording to fit your personal circumstances.

Fear and Anxiety

Some levels of fear and anxiety can be healthy. Fear can protect you from danger, while healthy levels of anxiety can help you be organized and ready for anything bad that may happen.

However, when fear is unfounded or irrational and affects your daily life, it needs to be addressed. It could potentially undermine your physical and emotional health.

Today, many people worldwide suffer from different types of phobias, such as fear of spiders, fear of war, fear of socializing, fear of heights, etc.

Phobia is an excessive fear or irrationality for certain objects or situations. People with a phobia usually do everything they can to avoid the stimulus that triggers their fear.

How to manage fear and anxiety with the help of EFT and Tapping

If you suffer from fear, phobias, or anxiety, and if traditional techniques haven't worked for you, you should try EFT, which has helped me overcome these disorders.

Tapping to deal with fear and anxiety

Rate your level of anxiety/fear on a scale of 1-10 (a rate of 10 denotes that the problem is more difficult to address).

Identify at what point you began to develop this fear.

In the latter case, you can frame the tapping script as "Even though I don't know the cause of the fear, I still accept and love myself."

Try to visualize the situation that triggers the anxiety/fear in your mind.

Use an EFT tapping script based on your situation to help you overcome the fear or anxiety.

"Even though I have this anxiety most of the time, I accept how I feel and still love myself."

Remember that you should be touching your karate cut point as you recite this.

Then touch the other points on your body, starting with the top of your head and working downward, and use a reminder phrase such as "I have this anxiety."

Rate your level of anxiety again (on a scale of 1-10, where a rate of 10 denotes that the problem is more difficult to deal with).

Assess how your level of anxiety compares before practicing tapping.

You may need to repeat the tapping process a couple of times, depending on the intensity of the problem.

Anxiety script

After you finish tapping and recite the setup phrase such as "Even though I have this anxiety most of the time, I accept how I feel and still love myself," you can use the following script to tap instead of using the reminder phrase.

For it to be more effective, replace the phrases with your thoughts and feelings.

Here is a script to start implementing the theory.

EFT Round 1: Expressing Anxiety
  Top of Head
These anxious feelings I have

Eyebrow
They are hard to live with
Side of the eye
There is something I have to do
Under the eye
But this anxiety leaves me paralyzed
Under the nose
It hinders my success
Chin
It paralyzes me and leaves me afraid
Collarbone
If you want to try new things, try new places
Under my arm
Or meet new people

EFT Round 2: Understanding Anxiety
Top of head
I know these feelings
Eyebrow
They should protect me and prepare me
Side of the eye
But they're just limiting me
Under the eye
They are leaving me afraid
Under my nose
I find it hard to let go
Chin

The more I think about my anxiety, the more it grows

Collarbone

Is there something wrong with me?

Under my arm

What can I change?

EFT Round 3: Explore the possibilities

Top of head

Focusing on anxiety is making things worse

Eyebrow

Continuing to focus on what will go wrong

Side of Eye

These thoughts are in my head

Under my eyes

And they start with me

Under the nose

If I can shift my attention

Chin

And my attention

Collarbone

To something more positive

Under the arm

I can create more positive thoughts

EFT Case 4: Relaxing

Top of head

I just need to breathe

Eyebrow

And regain my composure

Side of the eye

These thoughts are in my head

Under my eyes

Start with me

Under the nose

I will focus on feeling calm

Chin

And relaxed

Collarbone

Slower I inhale and exhale

Under Arm

The more relaxed I feel

EFT Round 5: Slowing down

Top of head

I just need to slow things down

Eyebrow

When I am calm and clear

Side of the eye

I will be able to perform better

Under the eye

Because my worries and anguish

Under the nose

Will disappear

Chin

Now I will slow down and relax

Collarbone

This anxiety is not helping me

Underarm

I have much more control when I am calm and relaxed

EFT Round 6: Choosing calm and clarity

Top of head

I choose to release this anxious energy

Eyebrow

And aim for a positive outcome

Side of the eye

When I let go of these fears and doubts

Under the eye

I will be able to succeed to a greater extent

Under the nose

When I am relaxed and focused

Chin

I can do and achieve anything

Collarbone

I choose to feel good about myself, knowing I'm smart and responsible.

Under Arm

I choose to feel calm, confident, and powerful

OK, let's move on to a script to help deal with specific phobias.

Script Phobia

After you finish tapping and recite the setup phrase such as "Even though I have this fear of needles, I accept how I feel and still love myself," you can use the following script to tap instead of using the reminder phrase.

Of course, to be more effective, you should replace the phrases with your thos and feelings.

EFT Round 1: *Express the phobia*

Top of Head

This phobia I have

Eyebrow

It is difficult to live with

Side of the eye

It makes me feel embarrassed

Under-eye

It is difficult to talk to people about

Under the nose

It makes going to the doctors a scary experience

Chin

Afraid I will faint

Collarbone

And creates a scene

Under the arm

And embarrasses me further

EFT Round 2: *Understanding the Phobia*

Top of head
I know this feeling
Eyebrow
It should protect and prepare me
Side of the eye
But it's just limiting me
Under the eye
It's leaving me afraid
Under the nose
To receive important medical care
Chin
Or donate blood for a good cause
Collarbone
I don't think anyone else I know has that problem.
Under the arm
What can I change?

EFT Round 3: Explore the possibilities

Top of head
Focus on the negative outcome
Eyebrow
It's just adding power to my fear
Side of the eye
Every time I stay a check
Under the eye
Because of fear
Under the nose

I reinforce this fear even more

Chin

If I can change my focus

Collarbone

Towards a more positive outcome

Under Arm

So I can create more positive thoughts and reduce fear

EFT Round 4: Relaxing

Top of head

I just need to breathe

Eyebrow

And regain my composure

Side of the eye

These thoughts that are in my head

Under my eyes

Start with me

Under the nose

There is nothing to fear

Chin

Nothing bad will happen

Collarbone

I just need to breathe in and out

Under my arm

And allow my mind to become more relaxed

EFT Round 5: Slowing down

Top of head
I just need to slow things down
Eyebrow
When I am calm and relaxed
Side of the eye
I can focus more on a positive outcome
Under the eye
Which will allow my worries
Under the nose
To disappear
Chin
Now I will slow down and relax
Collarbone
This fear is not helping me
Under my arm
It's in my way

EFT Round 6: Choosing calm and confidence

Top of Head
I choose to release this scary energy
Eyebrow
And aim for a positive outcome
Side of the eye
When I let go of these fears and doubts
Under the eye
I will become more confident
Under the nose

When I am relaxed and confident

Chin

I can do and achieve anything

Collarbone

I decided to feel good knowing that I am braver Arm

I choose to feel calm, confident and powerful

Depression or depressive thoughts

Today, depression is affecting more and more people, especially in the Western world. It can make us feel empty, sad, and hopeless, which drastically reduces our happiness in life.

Depression is thought to block positive energy and deplete our willpower by leaving us unmotivated to do even the simplest daily tasks.

However, the use of EFT and tapping can help combat depression.

A good example of an EFT installation script that you can use if you suffer from depression would be, "Even though I am currently suffering from depression, I accept that I will be able to overcome this and do well in my life."

DEPRESSION SCRIPT

After you have finished tapping and reciting the setup phrase such as "Even though I feel depressed, I accept how I feel and still love myself," you can use the following script to tap instead of using the reminder phrase.

As always, feel free to replace the phrases with your thoughts and feelings to make them more personal and effective.

EFT Round 1: Expressing Depression

Top of Head

This sadness I have

Eyebrow

It is hard to live with

Side of my eye

It makes me feel hopeless

Under my eyes

It reals me down

Under the nose

It makes everything seem colorless

Chin

It's sapping my energy

Collarbone

And draining my happiness

Under the arm

It is difficult to open up about it

EFT Round 2: Understanding Depression

Top of head

What is causing this feeling?

Eyebrow

What is the source?
Side of the eye
Why is it affecting me?
Under the eye
This depression
Under the nose
It's robbing me of my happiness
Chin
And positivity
Collarbone
I don't need it
Under the arm
How can I fix the problem?

EFT Round 3: Explore the possibilities
Top of Head
I need to see the good in life
Eyebrow
And open myself to good opportunities
Side of the eye
With my mind and heart
Under my eyes
Though things seem hard to do
Under the nose
They will be easier with time
Chin
If I can change my focus and attitude

Collarbone

Towards a more positive outcome

Under Arm

Then I can live life more fully

EFT Round 4: Opening

Top of head

I am willing

Eyebrow

To listen and try new things

Side of the eye

I am willing

Under the eye

To get on with my life

Under the nose

And leave this sadness behind

Chin

No use at all

Collarbone

Only drains me

Under my arm

My future can be bright again

EFT Round 5: Choosing Confidence and Hope

Top of Head

I choose to release this negative energy

Eyebrow

And aim for a positive outcome

Side of the eye
When I let go of this sadness and negativity
Under the eye
I will become more confident and hopeful
Under the nose
When I am confident and hopeful
Chin
I will become re-energized with life again
Collarbone
Positivity and energy will replace my depression
Under Arm
I will live a good and happy life
Next steps

OK, so you've read through the scripts and probably identified which one you think is probably best for you.

To experience the change and start seeing the benefits, you need to make a decision.

That is, to start tapping.

At first, this may seem strange. But, with persistence, you can start to feel calmer and more in control of your emotions.

To feel the benefit, we recommend setting aside to tap regularly.

Making tapping a habit becomes more of a band-aid or patch to use when your emotions get the better of you or spillover.

If you haven't started yet, when can you set aside 5-10 minutes for your first tapping session?

Once you start to feel the benefits, can you set aside some time each day to review the script you feel is most appropriate for that day?

Why not start today?

Chapter Seven
GAIN ENERGY
EFT Tapping for energy

*E*veryday life can be hectic and stressful. When you're busy, may find yourself lacking energy and feeling fatigued.

The following EFT tapping sequence is meant to help you rebalance your energy system. It will give you a rapid burst of energy and help you become more alive and alert. If you do this exercise daily, it will also increase your overall energy level.

How does EFT work to overcome fatigue?

To understand how EFT works to overcome fatigue and gain energy, it's important to go through the tapping points one by one. We will use four tapping points that are directly related to the body's energy system for this exercise. These are:

1. Under the eyes on the cheekbones
2. The collarbone
3. The thymus point or the center of the chest, and
4. The neurolymphatic points of the spleen
5. Under the eyes to stay grounded and connected to your rhythm

It is a society that creates a schedule for us to follow. This allows us to conform but also against our natural rhythm, which stresses and wears us down.

The Stomach Meridian is the pathway of energy and flows from around the eyes down the front of the body and legs to the second finger. The tapping point that hits the stomach meridian is located under the eyes on the cheekbones.

When energy flows smoothly through this meridian, you feel much more connected to the energies of the earth. This puts your body in perfect rhythm. When you touch these acupressure points, your energy becomes more grounded and guides your hormones to support your body's natural rhythm.

In terms of psycho-energy, when your body is in its natural rhythm, it can metabolize better. It also helps you become more adaptable to things you find difficult to adjust to. Reaching your natural rhythm will make you feel more stable and grounded so that you can go with the natural flow.

2. Collarbone to encourage a forward direction in energy flow

If you get tired even when you're just walking forward, it's a definite sign that you should pay more attention to these meridian points. These acupressure points are located just below the collarbone or clavicle. To locate them, place your fingertips on the U-shaped notch above your sternum. Now move your fingertips to each side and about an inch downward. You may feel a small depression here.

This is where the renal meridians end. The energy pathways of the renal meridians begin under the ball of the foot, moving up the inside of the leg, traveling to the front of the body, and finding its end at the collarbone.

By touching these points, which are also known as "K-27 points," you encourage the flow of energy to move in a forward direction by passing through all of your meridians. This helps to kick-start your energy system, making you feel more energetic and alert.

3. The thymus or the center of the chest to obtain vital energy

Dr. John Diamond, who wrote Life Energy, points out that the thymus gland is responsible for controlling the body's vital energy. This gland is located just below the top of the sternum in the center of the chest. He's got an enormous part to play in the immune system. This is exactly what Tarzan beats before he gets an instant boost of energy.

4. The neurolymphatic points of the spleen to eliminate toxins and assimilate Change

As part of the lymphatic system, these points help flush toxins from the body. These points are the depression located between the 7th and 8th ribs. It is located just below the level of the sternum or breastbone. To locate these points, move your fingertips under your breasts in line with your nipples. Then move them to lower just above the next rib.

You can eliminate toxins and regulate hormones and blood chemistry by tapping, not touching, these points. Performing this exercise also helps fight infections and promote healthy food metabolism. It is also known to help relieve stress and dizziness. Also, if you want to initiate a change in a specific aspect of your life, the meridian energy of the spleen is what you need to work on.

Touch sequence and energy instructions

Suppose you feel pain in these points; massage or rub them before you begin with touch. As you work on these acupressure points, be sure to breathe deeply through your nose and exhale slowly through your mouth. If possible, take three deep breaths as you perform each step. Feel free to do more if necessary.

Under your eyes, "I am joined to the earth. I feel rooted. I am finding my natural rhythm."

Take deep breaths. As you touch and repeat these affirmations, imagine the energy traveling from under your eyes to your cheekbones, going up around your eyes, going to the front of your torso, down to your legs, and ending your foot right at your second toe.

Collarbone: "I am balanced and centered. I am moving forward gracefully with my life."

Visualize the energy flowing from under your foot to the inside of your legs, traveling higher in front of your body and terminating on the meridian points you are touching.

Chest center: "My life energy is remarkable. I am filled with love, faith, courage, gratitude, and trust."

Begin by raising your hand to make a fist. Then, start tapping the center of your chest as Tarzan does. Take deep breaths and repeat these affirmations.

Neurolymphatic Spleen Points: "Change is always good. I'm moving with the flow gracefully."

Touch below the breast in the ribs. Breathe deeply and repeat these touch statements.

Chapter Eight
HOW TO YOU TAPPING TODAY

In our hectic daily lives, there are emotional issues common to all. With the pressures of personal finance,

keeping up with friends and family, and being constantly on the go, it's easy to see how people can feel lost and discouraged in modern life.

EFT can give you the power to eliminate emotional issues that affect your mindset and daily performance.

Let's be honest for a moment. How often did you feel a bit out of control in the last week? More often than we'd like to say probably.

We all feel the pressure of fast-paced modern life, but if we let our emotions get control of us, situations can quickly spiral out of control.

Start by using EFT in your daily routine whenever

your emotions start to take over. By tapping, you can help yourself feel safer, more confident, and more self-aware so you can keep moving forward with your day.

Here are seven of the most common daily applications of tapping.

1. *Anger*

Anger, frustration, stress, annoyance, and all the associated emotions can make up a large part of today's hectic life.

Maybe for you, it's a difficult relative, a child, a boss or co-worker, or even road rage that makes you angry.

Feeling like your space has been violated or offended will bring up negative, angry feelings that can change your mood and day.

Here is an example of how EFT changed Andy's life:

Before Andy used EFT, the smallest of offenses would set him off. Andy had a closed, self-preserving view of the world where everyone could be out to get him at any time!

So every time someone pushed in line, passed him on the highway, or spoke bluntly, he was angry that he wasn't being treated fairly. After this anger, it would take hours before he could return to a normal state of mind.

With EFT, Andy was able to ease his frustrations

and cool his anger to get on with his day. Before he knew it, what had angered Andy would slip away like water off a duck's back.

He discovered that anger is no better retaliation than overcoming it and moving on with your day!

Learning how to overcome anger is something you can do with EFT.

When you touch on the sequence, it is helpful to acknowledge and explicitly state what set you off.

Try this and some of these other phrases to curb feelings of frustration:

- I am angry at my {spouse, child, coworker, etc.}
- I am frustrated and angry
- This anger will keep me from doing what I need to do
- I can't afford this anger
- This anger, I can let it go

2. *Impatience*

With our booming economies and globalization, it's not a long stretch to have to wait everywhere we want to serve.

There are queues at the checkout, queues on the

phone, queues to get into toilets, restaurants, queues in traffic - there is simply no way to escape the wait.

Impatience is that itchy feeling when you need something right away. And oh boy, does it suck when you're engulfed in nothing but impatience.

Here's an example of how EFT changed Sue's life, in her own words:

"I can attest that one area of my life where I struggled with impatience was online shopping.

I would spend hours and days browsing online stores, comparing patterns, and considering exchange rates and shipping prices to find the perfect purchase.

It wasn't until after I paid that I realized it would take over a week to get the item into my hot little hands. More than a week...outrageous!

If the package arrived when I wasn't home, it would be another day to pick it up from the post office. In the week that the package would be in transit, I would wait impatiently, agitated, and not in a good mood.

Impatience controlled me!"

If you find impatience in your life, here are some EFT touch phrases you can use.

- I feel impatient, but that's okay
- I want (what I want) now, but I can wait
- I still have one more day to move forward

- I won't let impatience stop me from my day
- My life will go on while I wait

3. *Worry*

With the convenience of modern life, we all feel like we are under pressure.

All this pressure leads to a very stressful 21st-century life! Things were not as fast as they were a couple of decades ago.

Now we have to worry about the looming specter of redundancy, our ability to pay our bills, and the physical and financial security of ourselves and our loved ones.

When worry plagues the mind, the action takes a back seat. Worry hijacks our emotional centers, shakes the fundamental foundations of our being.

How can you take risks when all you're worried about are negative outcomes? How can you enjoy life when all there is, is the danger? These are the pitfalls of a problematic life.

These are some of the things Harry had to say about his experience of living with worry:

I know how much worry can control your life. I used to worry about my financial situation all the time. Several years ago, I moved for work, away from family and friends.

Shortly after that, the company I worked for hit hard

times, leaving me worrying every day about my job, my livelihood, my rent, and my bills.

Worry kept me from exploring alternative avenues to make money.

It wasn't until Harry touched EFT that he overcame his worries, free himself from the paycheck and become the writer and lifestyle coach he is today!

With the Emotional Freedom Technique, you can minimize your worries to start taking those risks that will help you achieve emotional freedom.

Here are some EFT touch phrases you can use:

- I am worried about my situation
- I know what I want, but the worry is stopping me
- I can overcome my worry
- I will not let worry stop me from taking action
- I am confident and feel secure in myself

4. Low self-esteem

Low self-esteem is one of the biggest problems people face every day.

Modern life dangles the image of perfection in front of us with every sitcom, movie, reality show, commercial, and magazine.

Physically, magazines demand that we have the "perfect abs" or the "firm butt" to get the man or woman we want.

Advertisements sell us lifestyles we can only dream of, being the envy of family and friends with a great new home, driving down rolling hills in our newest SUVs, being successful with a new watch or fragrance... the list could go on!

The main message these images sell to you and me is that we are not good enough as we are right now.

Unfortunately, the ads aren't going away anytime soon, but there is a way we can preserve our self-esteem when that nagging feeling emerges. Yes, you guessed it, I touch EFT!

Low self-esteem can also stem from bad self-perceptions within ourselves. These self-perceptions are often borrowed from childhood or some other twisted source. And the truth is, they are simply not true.

It is proven repeatedly that we can be harder on ourselves when it comes to self-esteem.

However, as a free-thinking, self-directed adult, you can now begin to address your false self-perceptions through eFT.

Try using these phrases whenever low self-esteem tries to creep into your life:

- I don't feel confident in my skin
- I feel like I need to change, but I'm perfect the way I am now
- I'm happy with my life and myself
- I decide what I need in my life
- I have the self-esteem I need

5. *Restlessness*

Restlessness and lack of sleep is a huge problem in our modern society.

Work has started to follow people home with the mainstreaming of the internet and smartphones. Carbonated energy drinks, caffeine pills, tea, coffee, alarm clocks, fatigue, and being on edge are all symptoms that we, as a culture, have given away valuable sleep in exchange for busy schedules.

So what happens when our head hits the pillow at the end of a busy day?

Well, if you're anything like me over the day, you're tossing and turning, feeling restless, be aware of every second that passes and think about what still needs to be done.

Modern life makes it hard to fall asleep! But with

the Emotional Freedom Technique, you may find it easier to rest at night.

EFT can help you calm your nervous system and quiet your mind to rest properly.

When you touch your restlessness, try these additional techniques:

Breathe deeply and consciously

Tighten your eyelids closed and with your eyeballs, direct them upward and inward toward the center of your forehead. This activates alpha waves in the brain for deep relaxation.

When you open your eyes, focus them on a point in the distance, out the window, or on the roof.

After these additional techniques, you can use EFT to tap away from restlessness. Try these mantras or variations to put them to sleep quickly!

- I feel restless
- But my body and mind feel active.
- This restlessness means I will not sleep
- I need a relaxing and restful sleep
- I permit myself to sleep

6. *Fear of success or failure*

The fear of achievement and the fear of failure is the biggest negative blocks to achieving the life we desire.

Here is something from Paul's story:

For years I marked the terror of quitting my job to start my own business. I was too scared about the consequences of failure in my business idea.

I often asked, "What would it mean for me if my business failed?" and "What would others think if I failed?"

And on the flip side, the fear of success kept me in a daily grind: "What would I do with all that money?", "Success is not for me. After all, I only come from a middle-class, working-class background."

Fear led me into a state of stasis where I was only happy to receive a consistent monthly check.

It wasn't until I learned about taking control of the fear of failure and success that I was able to step away from my passive attitude, "go with the flow," and direct my life.

If you fear failure or success, you need to evaluate your beliefs about failure, money, and business.

Look back into your childhood and past to see where these beliefs were formed. If there are negative emotions there, those are the ones you can target!

Blast those negative feelings with some EFT phrases:

- I am afraid of failure/success

- I feel I don't deserve success/failure is not acceptable
- Failure is not defeat/Success is not bad

7. Procrastination

Perhaps the most negative use of time in our modern lives is when procrastination takes over.

I bet you've been there too; 10 minutes of television ends up being 30 minutes, And before you realize it, your entire night is over!

Or you wake up in the morning and waste half an hour or an hour just checking your social media before you even get out of bed.

Technology is at the center of our lives. And although technology has increased our productivity and efficiency, our easy access to the internet has made procrastination much easier, making us less productive!

If we're not careful, a little 'break' at our computers to read the news, watch a movie, or check social media ends up wasting a whole hour or maybe much more!

What's worse is that when we procrastinate, the time spent is often not even very pleasant.

Time spent procrastinating is different than time spent in active mental engagement with hobbies or activities.

How many times did you believe that? Relaxingor

unwinding when you were just wasting valuable time? Ask yourself, do you feel better after procrastinating?

I guess the answer is not - it's just something we do without really thinking about it.

Procrastination doesn't help us take action necessary for the life we love; it's not fun and makes us feel good.

Whatever the reason you procrastinate, there is little to suggest happy, successful people procrastinate all the time.

It is action, not procrastination, that makes the world go round.

It's also an action that will help you achieve the emotional freedom you deserve.

Stop procrastinating in its tracks with these EFT phrases ... Now!

- I accept that I want to procrastinate
- I know that procrastination is unproductive
- I can let go of this feeling to procrastinate
- I am in control of my time
- I know what I need to do

We looked at seven different ways to use touch to help manage and control your emotions.

These emotions included anger, impatience, worry,

low self-esteem, restlessness, fear of success or failure, and procrastination.

To get the most benefit from this book, go back and underline or highlight those sections you believe will be very helpful.

That way, you'll have them ready for the next time you start to feel your emotions slipping away from you.

Chapter Nine
CONCLUSIONS

The emotional Freedom Technique has gained a reputation around the world. Millions of people use EFT for a happier, healthier, and more balanced life. Will EFT tapping live up to its promise for you too? There's no other way to find out than to try it.

Use the information you learned in this book to improve your condition or resolve any emotional or internal conflict you may experience or issues you may encounter. Use it to improve your life. Take advantage of EFT to be more positive and happier!

Happy Tapping!

www.ingramcontent.com/pod-product-compliance
Lightning Source LLC
Chambersburg PA
CBHW071116030426
42336CB00013BA/2115